Keto Diet For Beginners

Proven Strategies On How You Can Get The Most Out Of The Ketogenic Diet With Easy & Delicious Recipes To Reactivate Your Genes Of Health, Energy, And Burn Fat

Written By

Winifred Campbell

Table of Contents

INTRODUCTION

Thank you for purchasing this book!

The ketogenic diet can help you from this point of view, eliminating carbohydrates and promoting the elimination of fats from our body. Another advantage is its flexibility, in fact, you can play with macros and adapt them to your needs and the way you live, in addition to the progress made, of course.

Start gradually, your body has adapted for years to an unhealthy lifestyle, so do not overdo it overnight. Take your time and slowly reach your goals. There is no need to run, this is a marathon, not 100 meters.

At first, you may feel tired, tired, without energy. Don't worry it's a normal thing, it's your body that is adapting to the new food style. You're taking away its basic source of energy, carbohydrates, it's logical that it has to adapt. It must change the main energy source, it must switch to using fats, but this takes time, two or three days are necessary. The drop in sugars could decrease your pressure for a couple of days, avoid exercise and there will be no problems. The resulting benefits will be enormous.

Enjoy your reading!

Shrimp Curry

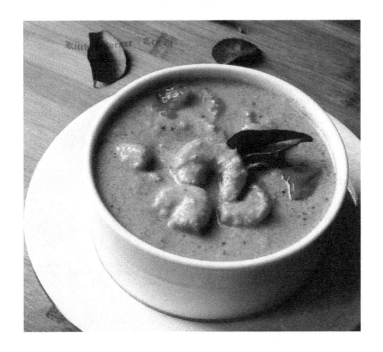

Preparation Time: 15 Minutes

Cooking Time: 21 Minutes

Servings: 4

Ingredients:

- 2 tablespoons coconut oil

- ½ of yellow onion, minced

- 2 garlic cloves, minced

- 1 teaspoon ground turmeric

- 1 teaspoon ground cumin

- 1 teaspoon paprika

- 1 (14-ounce) can unsweetened coconut milk

- 1 large tomato, chopped finely

- Salt, as required

- 1 pound shrimp, peeled and deveined

- 2 tablespoons fresh cilantro, chopped

Direction:

1. Melt coconut oil in a large wok over medium heat and sauté the onion for about 5 minutes.

2. Add the garlic, and spices, and sauté for about 1 minute.

3. Add the coconut milk, tomato, and salt, and bring to a gentle boil.

4. Lower the heat to low and simmer for about 10 minutes, stirring occasionally.

5. Stir in the shrimp and cilantro and simmer for about 4–5 minutes.

6. Remove the wok from heat and serve hot.

Nutrition:

- **Calories:** 168 Cal

- **Fat:** 15g

- **Carbs:** 5 g

- **Protein:** 9 g

- **Fiber:** 7 g

Seafood Stew

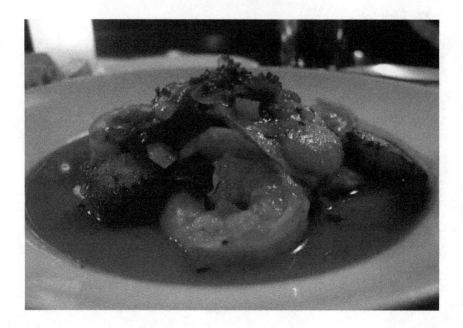

Preparation Time: 20 Minutes

Cooking Time: 30 Minutes

Servings: 8

Ingredients:

- 2 tablespoons butter

- 1 medium yellow onion, chopped

- 2 garlic cloves, minced

- 1 Serrano pepper, chopped

- ¼ teaspoon red pepper flakes, crushed

- ½ pound fresh tomatoes, chopped

- 1½ cups homemade fish broth

- 1 pound red snapper fillets, cubed

- ½ pound shrimp, peeled and deveined

- ¼ pound fresh squid, cleaned and cut into rings

- ¼ pound bay scallops

- ¼ pound mussels

- 2 tablespoons fresh lime juice

- ½ cup fresh basil, chopped

Direction:

1. In a large soup pan, melt butter over medium heat and sauté the onion for about 5–6 minutes.

2. Add the garlic, Serrano pepper, and red pepper flakes, and sauté for about 1 minute.

3. Add tomatoes and broth and bring to a gentle simmer.

4. Reduce the heat and cook for about 10 minutes.

5. Add the tilapia and cook for about 2 minutes.

6. Stir in the remaining seafood and cook for about 6–8 minutes.

7. Stir in the lemon juice, basil, salt, and black pepper, and remove from heat.

8. Serve hot.

Nutrition:

- **Calories:** 199 Cal

- **Fat:** 12.1 g

- **Carbs:** 7.5 g

- **Protein:** 8 g

- **Fiber:** 3 g

Tomato & Mozzarella Salad

Preparation Time: 15 Minutes

Cooking Time: 15 Minutes

Servings: 8

Ingredients:

- 4 cups cherry tomatoes, halved

- 1½ pounds mozzarella cheese, cubed

- ¼ cup fresh basil leaves, chopped

- ¼ cup olive oil

- 2 tablespoons fresh lemon juice

- 1 teaspoon fresh oregano, minced

- 1 teaspoon fresh parsley, minced

- 2–4 drops liquid stevia

- Salt and ground black pepper, as required

Direction:

1. In a salad bowl, mix together tomatoes, mozzarella, and basil.

2. In a small bowl, add remaining ingredients and beat until well combined.

3. Place dressing over salad and toss to coat well.

4. Serve immediately.

Nutrition:

Calories: 310 Cal

Fat: 18 g

Carbs: 7 g

Protein: 8 g

Fiber: 3 g

Cucumber & Tomato Salad

Preparation Time: 15 Minutes

Cooking Time: 15 Minutes

Servings: 8

Ingredients:

Salad:

- 3 large English cucumbers, thinly sliced

- 2 cups tomatoes, chopped

- 6 cups lettuce, torn

Dressing:

- 4 tablespoons olive oil

- 2 tablespoons balsamic vinegar

- 1 tablespoon fresh lemon juice

- Salt and ground black pepper, as required

Direction:

1. For salad: In a large bowl, add the cucumbers, onion, cucumbers, and mix.

2. For dressing: In a small bowl, add all the ingredients and beat until well combined.

3. Place the dressing over the salad and toss to coat well.

4. Serve immediately.

Nutrition:

- **Calories:** 268 Cal

- **Fat:** 18 g

- **Carbs:** 7 g

- **Protein**: 8 g

- **Fiber:** 3 g

Chicken & Broccoli Casserole

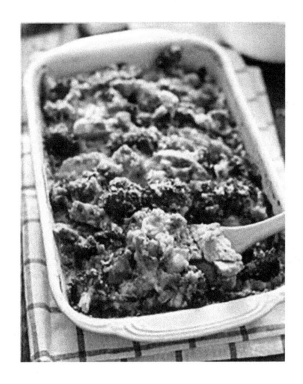

Preparation Time: 15 Minutes

Cooking Time: 35 Minutes

Servings: 6

Ingredients:

- 2 tablespoons butter

- ¼ cup cooked bacon, crumbled

- 2½ cups cheddar cheese, shredded and divided

- 4 ounces' cream cheese, softened

- ¼ cup heavy whipping cream

- ½ pack ranch seasoning mix

- 2/3 cup homemade chicken broth

- 1½ cups small broccoli florets

- 2 cups cooked grass-fed chicken breast, shredded

Direction:

1. Preheat your oven to 350°F.

2. Arrange a rack in the upper portion of the oven.

3. For chicken mixture: In a large wok, melt the butter over low heat.

4. Add the bacon, ½ cup of cheddar cheese, cream cheese, heavy whipping cream, ranch seasoning, and broth, and with a wire whisk, beat until well combined.

5. Cook for about 5 minutes, stirring frequently.

6. Meanwhile, in a microwave-safe dish, place the broccoli and microwave until desired tenderness is achieved.

7. In the wok, add the chicken and broccoli and mix until well combined.

8. Remove from the heat and transfer the mixture into a casserole dish.

9. Top the chicken mixture with the remaining cheddar cheese.

10. Bake for about 25 minutes.

11. Now, set the oven to broiler.

12. Broil the chicken mixture for about 2–3 minutes or until cheese is bubbly.

13. Serve hot.

Nutrition:

- **Calories:** 168 Cal

- **Fat:** 19 g

- **Carbs:** 8 g

- **Protein:** 10 g

- **Fiber:** 5 g

Turkey Chili

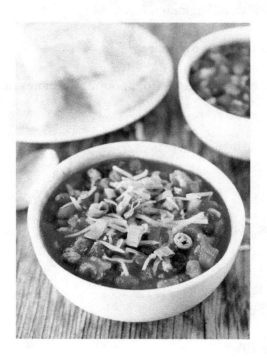

Preparation Time: 15 Minutes

Cooking Time: 120 Minutes

Servings: 8

Ingredients:

- 2 tablespoons olive oil

- 1 small yellow onion, chopped

- 1 green bell pepper, seeded and chopped

- 4 garlic cloves, minced

- 1 jalapeño pepper, chopped

- 1 teaspoon dried thyme, crushed

- 2 tablespoons red chili powder

- 1 tablespoon ground cumin

- 2 pounds lean ground turkey

- 2 cups fresh tomatoes, chopped finely

- 2 ounces' sugar-free tomato paste

- 2 cups homemade chicken broth

- 1 cup of water

- Salt and ground black pepper, as required

- 1 cup cheddar cheese, shredded

Direction:

1. In a large Dutch oven, heat oil over medium heat and sauté the onion and bell pepper for about 5–7 minutes.

2. Add the garlic, jalapeño pepper, thyme, and spices and sauté for about 1 minute.

3. Add the turkey and cook for about 4–5 minutes.

4. Stir in the tomatoes, tomato paste, and cacao powder, and cook for about 2 minutes.

5. Add in the broth and water and bring to a boil.

6. Now, reduce the heat to low and simmer, covered for about 2 hours.

7. Add in salt and black pepper and remove from the heat.

8. Top with cheddar cheese and serve hot.

Nutrition:

1. **Calories:** 308 Cal

2. **Fat:** 20 g

3. **Carbs:** 10 g

4. **Protein:** 8 g

5. **Fiber:** 3 g

Beef Curry

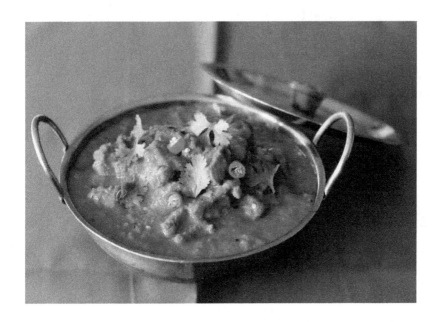

Preparation Time: 10 Minutes

Cooking Time: 205 Minutes

Servings: 8

Ingredients:

- 2 tablespoons butter

- 2 tomatoes, chopped finely

- 2 tablespoons curry powder

- 2½ cups unsweetened coconut milk

- ½ cup homemade chicken broth

- 2½ pounds grass-fed beef chuck roast, cubed into 1-inch size

- Salt and ground black pepper, as required

- ¼ cup fresh cilantro, chopped

Direction:

1. Melt butter in a big pan over low heat and cook the tomatoes and curry powder for about 3–4 minutes, crushing the tomatoes with the back of spoon.

2. Stir in the coconut milk, and broth, and bring to a gentle simmer, stirring occasionally.

3. Simmer for about 4–5 minutes.

4. Stir in beef and bring to a boil over medium heat.

5. Adjust the heat to low and cook, covered for about 2½ hours, stirring occasionally

6. Remove from heat and with a slotted spoon, transfer the beef into a bowl.

7. Set the pan of curry aside for about 10 minutes.

8. With a slotted spoon, remove the fats from top of curry.

9. Return the pan over medium heat.

10. Stir in the cooked beef and bring to a gentle simmer.

11. Adjust the heat to low and cook, uncovered for about 30 minutes, or until desired thickness.

12. Stir in salt and black pepper and remove from the heat.

13. Garnish with fresh cilantro and serve hot.

Nutrition:

- **Calories:** 360 Cal
- **Fat:** 25 g
- **Carbs:** 3 g
- **Protein:** 18 g
- **Fiber:** 3 g

Shepherd's Pie

Preparation Time: 20 Minutes

Cooking Time: 50 Minutes

Servings: 6

Ingredients:

- ¼ cup olive oil

- 1 pound grass-fed ground beef

- ½ cup celery, chopped

- ¼ cup yellow onion, chopped

- 3 garlic cloves, minced

- 1 cup tomatoes, chopped

- 2 (12-ounce) packages riced cauliflower, cooked and well-drained

- 1 cup cheddar cheese, shredded

Direction:

1. Preheat your oven to 350°F.

2. Heat oil in a large nonstick wok over medium heat and cook the ground beef, celery, onions, and garlic for about 8–10 minutes.

3. Remove from the heat and drain the excess grease.

4. Immediately stir in the tomatoes.

5. Transfer mixture into a 10x7-inch casserole dish evenly.

6. In a food processor, add the cauliflower, cheeses, cream, and thyme, and pulse until a mashed potatoes-like mixture is formed.

7. Spread the cauliflower mixture over the meat in the casserole dish evenly.

8. Bake for about 35–40 minutes.

9. Remove casserole dish from oven and let it cool slightly before serving.

10. Cut into desired sized pieces and serve.

Nutrition:

- **Calories:** 404 Cal

- **Fat:** 19 g

- **Carbs:** 10 g

- **Protein:** 19 g

- **Fiber:**5 g

Pork with Veggies

Preparation Time: 15 Minutes

Cooking Time: 15 Minutes

Servings: 5

Ingredients:

- 1 quid pork loin, cut into thin strips

- 2 tablespoons olive oil, divided

- 1 teaspoon garlic, minced

- 1 teaspoon fresh ginger, minced

- 2 tablespoons low-sodium soy sauce

- 1 tablespoon fresh lemon juice

- 1 teaspoon sesame oil

- 1 tablespoon granulated erythritol

- 1 teaspoon arrowroot star

- 10 ounces' broccoli florets

- 1 carrot, peeled and sliced

- 1 big red bell pepper, seeded and cut into strips

- 2 scallions, cut into 2-inch pieces

Direction:

1. In a bowl, mix well pork strips, ½ tablespoon of olive oil, garlic, and ginger.

2. For the sauce: Add the soy sauce, lemon juice, sesame oil, Swerve, and arrowroot starch in a small bowl and mix well.

3. Heat the remaining olive oil in a big nonstick wok over high heat and sear the pork strips for about 3–4 minutes or until cooked through.

4. With a slotted spoon, transfer the pork into a bowl.

5. In the same wok, add the carrot and cook for about 2–3 minutes.

6. Add the broccoli, bell pepper, and scallion, and cook, covered for about 1–2 minutes.

7. Stir the cooked pork, sauce, and stir fry, and cook for about 3–5 minutes or until desired doneness, stirring occasionally.

8. Remove from the heat and serve.

Nutrition:

- **Calories:** 268 Cal

- **Fat:** 18 g

- **Carbs:** 7 g

- **Protein:** 8 g

- **Fiber:** 3 g

Pork Taco Bake

Preparation Time: 15 Minutes

Cooking Time: 60 Minutes

Servings: 6

Ingredients:

Crust

- 3 organic eggs

- 4 ounces' cream cheese, softened

- ½ teaspoon taco seasoning

- 1/3 cup heavy cream

- 8 ounces' cheddar cheese, shredded

Topping:

- 1 pound lean ground pork

- 4 ounces canned chopped green chilies

- ¼ cup sugar-free tomato sauce

- 3 teaspoons taco seasoning

- 8 ounces' cheddar cheese, shredded

- ¼ cup fresh basil leaves

Direction:

1. Preheat your oven to 375°F.

2. Lightly grease a 13x9-inch baking dish.

3. For crust: In a bowl, add the eggs and cream cheese, and beat until well combined and smooth.

4. Add the taco seasoning and heavy cream, and mix well.

5. Place cheddar cheese evenly in the bottom of prepared baking dish.

6. Spread cream cheese mixture evenly over cheese.

7. Bake for about 25–30 minutes.

8. Remove baking dish from the oven and set aside for about 5 minutes.

9. Meanwhile, for the topping: Heat a large nonstick wok over medium-high heat and cook the pork for about 8–10 minutes.

10. Drain the excess grease from wok.

11. Stir in the green chilies, tomato sauce, and taco seasoning, and remove from the heat.

12. Place the pork mixture evenly over crust and sprinkle with cheese.

13. Bake for about 18–20 minutes or until bubbly.

14. Remove from the oven and set aside for about 5 minutes.

15. Cut into desired size slices and serve with the garnishing of basil leaves.

Nutrition:

- **Calories:** 198 Cal

- **Fat:** 12 g

- **Carbs:** 8 g

- **Protein:** 19 g

- **Fiber:** 3 g

Shrimp Lettuce Wraps

Preparation Time: 20 Minutes

Cooking Time: 4 Minutes

Servings: 6

Ingredients:

Shrimp:

- 1 teaspoon olive oil

- 2 pounds' shrimp, peeled, deveined, and chopped

- ½ teaspoon ground cumin

- 1 teaspoon red chili powder

- Salt and ground black pepper, to taste

Wraps:

- 1 cup tomato, chopped finely

- ½ cup onion, chopped

- 2 tablespoons fresh parsley, chopped

- 12 butter lettuce leaves

Direction:

1. For shrimp: In a large wok, heat the oil over medium heat and cook the shrimp, spices, salt, and black pepper for about 3–4 minutes.

2. Remove the wok from the heat and set aside to cool slightly.

3. Meanwhile, in a bowl, mix together tomato, onion, and parsley.

4. Arrange the lettuce leaves onto serving plates.

5. Divide the shrimp over lettuce leaves evenly.

6. Top with tomato mixture evenly and serve.

Nutrition:

- **Calories:** 199 Cal

- **Fat:** 18 g

- **Carbs:** 4 g

- **Protein:** 9 g

- **Fiber:** 5 g

Chicken Stuffed Avocado

Preparation Time: 15 Minutes

Cooking Time: 0 Minutes

Servings: 2

Ingredients:

- 1 cup grass-fed cooked chicken, shredded

- 1 avocado, halved and pitted

- 1 tablespoon fresh lime juice

- ¼ cup yellow onion, chopped finely

- ¼ cup plain Greek yogurt

- 1 teaspoon Dijon mustard

- Pinch of cayenne pepper

- Salt and ground black pepper, to taste

Direction:

1. With a spoon, scoop out the flesh from the middle of each avocado half and transfer into a bowl.

2. Add the lime juice and mash until well combined.

3. Add remaining ingredients and stir to combine.

4. Divide the chicken mixture into avocado halves evenly and serve immediately.

Nutrition:

- **Calories:** 228 Cal

- **Fat:** 13 g

- **Carbs:** 9 g

- **Protein:** 10 g

- **Fiber:** 3 g

Chicken & Veggie Skewers

Preparation Time: 15 Minutes

Cooking Time: 8 Minutes

Servings: 6

Ingredients:

- ¼ cup parmesan cheese, grated

- 3 tablespoons olive oil

- 2 garlic cloves, minced

- 1 cup fresh basil leaves, chopped

- Salt and ground black pepper, to taste

- 1¼ pounds grass-fed boneless, skinless chicken breast, cut into 1-inch cubes

- 1 large green bell pepper, seeded and cubed

- 24 cherry tomatoes

Direction:

1. Add cheese, butter, garlic, basil, salt, and black pepper in a food processor and pulse until smooth.

2. Transfer the basil mixture into a large bowl.

3. Add the chicken cubes and mix well.

4. Cover the bowl and refrigerate to marinate for at least 4–5 hours.

5. Preheat the grill to medium-high heat. Generously, grease the grill grate.

6. Strand the chicken, bell pepper cubes, and tomatoes onto presoaked woody skewers.

7. Place the skewers onto the grill and cook for about 6–8 minutes, flipping occasionally.

8. Remove from the grill and place onto a plate for about 5 minutes before serving.

Nutrition:

- **Calories:** 201 Cal

- **Fat:** 19 g

- **Carbs:** 8 g

- **Protein:** 9 g

- **Fiber:** 4 g

Stuffed Tomatoes

Preparation Time: 15 Minutes

Cooking Time: 15 Minutes

Servings: 10

Ingredients:

- 1 pound gluten-free sausage, links removed and crumbled

- 10 medium tomatoes

- 3 tablespoons olive oil

- 10 thin Monterey Jack cheese slices

- ½ cup Monterey Jack cheese, shredded

- 2 tablespoons fresh chives, chopped finely

Direction:

1. Preheat the oven to 350°F.

2. Heat a lightly greased wok over medium heat and cook the sausage for about 6–8 minutes.

3. Eliminate from the heat and drain off any grease from sausage meat.

4. Carefully, cut a thin slice at the end of each tomato.

5. Now, cut the top part of each tomato and carefully, remove the core and seeds.

6. Coat the outer sides of tomatoes with oil lightly.

7. Arrange 1 cheese slice insides of each tomato and fill with cooked sausage.

8. Top with the shredded cheese.

9. Arrange the tomatoes onto a baking sheet.

10. Bake for approximately 5–8 minutes or until cheese is melted.

11. Remove the baking sheet from oven and set aside to cool for about 1–2 minutes before serving.

12. Garnish with chives and serve.

Nutrition:

- **Calories:** 198 Cal

- **Fat:** 18 g

- **Carbs:** 7 g

- **Protein:** 8 g

- **Fiber:** 3 g

Crab Cakes

Preparation Time: 15 Minutes

Cooking Time: 28 Minutes

Servings: 4

Ingredients:

Crab Cakes:

- 2 tablespoons olive oil, divided

- ½ cup onion, chopped finely

- 3 tablespoons blanched almond flour

- ¼ cup organic egg whites

- 2 tablespoons mayonnaise

- 1 tablespoon dried parsley, crushed

- 1 teaspoon yellow mustard

- 1 teaspoon Worcestershire sauce

- 1 tablespoon Old Bay seasoning

- Salt and ground black pepper, to taste

- 1 pound lump crabmeat, drained

Salad:

- 5 cups fresh baby arugula

- 2 tomatoes, chopped

- 2 tablespoons olive oil

- Salt and ground black pepper, to taste

Direction:

1. For crab cakes: Heat 2 teaspoons of olive oil in a wok over medium heat and sauté onion for about 8–10 minutes.

2. Remove the frying pan from heat and set aside to cool slightly.

3. Place cooked onion and remaining ingredients except for crabmeat in a mixing bowl and mix until well combined.

4. Add the crabmeat and mildly, stir to combine.

5. Make 8 equal-sized patties from the mixture.

6. Arrange the patties onto a foil-lined tray and refrigerate for about 30 minutes.

7. In a large frying pan, heat remaining oil over medium-low heat and cook patties in 2 batches for about 3–4 minutes per side or until desired doneness.

8. For salad: In a bowl, add all ingredients, and toss to coat well.

9. Divide salad onto serving plates and to each with 2 patties.

10. Serve immediately.

Nutrition:

- **Calories:** 268 Cal

- **Fat:** 18 g

- **Carbs:** 7 g

- **Protein:** 8 g

- **Fiber:** 3 g

Pepperoni Pizza

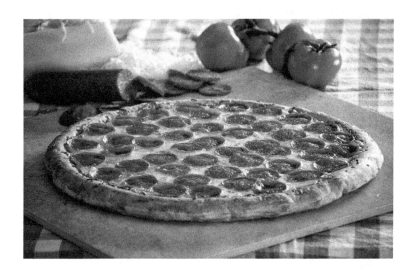

Preparation Time: 15 Minutes

Cooking Time: 20 Minutes

Servings: 8

Ingredients:

- 2 cups mozzarella cheese

- 1 large organic egg

- 3 tablespoons cream cheese, softened

- ¾ cup almond flour

- 1 tablespoon psyllium husk

- 1 tablespoon Italian seasoning

- Salt and ground black pepper, to taste

- 1 teaspoon butter, melted

Direction:

1. Preheat the oven to 400°F

2. For the crust: In a microwave-safe bowl, place mozzarella cheese and microwave on High for about 90 seconds or until melted completely.

3. In the bowl of mozzarella, add eggs and cream cheese and mix until well combined.

4. Add the remaining ingredients and mix until well combined and a dough ball forms.

5. Coat the dough ball with melted butter and place it onto a smooth surface.

6. With your hands, press the dough ball into a circle.

7. Arrange the crust onto a baking sheet and bake for approximately 10 minutes.

8. Carefully, flip the side and bake for approximately 2–4 minutes.

9. Remove the crust from oven.

10. Spread the tomato sauce over the crust evenly.

11. Arrange the pepperoni slices over tomato sauce evenly and sprinkle with cheese.

12. Bake for approximately 3–5 minutes.

13. Remove the pizza from oven and sprinkle with oregano.

14. Cut into 6 equal-sized wedges and serve.

Nutrition:

- **Calories:** 198 Cal

- **Fat:** 13 g

- **Carbs:** 7 g

- **Protein:** 8 g

- **Fiber:** 3 g

Bacon with Mushrooms

Preparation Time: 15 Minutes

Cooking Time: 16 Minutes

Servings: 2

Ingredients:

- 4 bacon slices, cut into ½-inch pieces

- 2 cups fresh mushrooms, sliced

- 1 tablespoon garlic, chopped

- 2 fresh thyme sprigs

Direction:

1. Heat a large cast-iron wok over medium heat and cook the bacon for about 5–6 minutes or until crispy.

2. Add the mushrooms and cook for about 4–5 minutes, stirring occasionally.

3. Stir in the garlic and thyme and cook for about 4–5 minutes, stirring occasionally.

4. Discard the thyme sprigs and serve hot.

Nutrition:

- **Calories:** 148 Cal

- **Fat:** 19 g

- **Carbs:** 7 g

- **Protein:** 10 g

- **Fiber:** 8 g

Shrimp with Zucchini Noodles

Preparation Time: 15 Minutes

Cooking Time: 7Minutes

Servings: 4

Ingredients:

- 2 tablespoons unsalted butter

- 1 large garlic clove, minced

- ¼ teaspoon red pepper flakes, crushed

- 1 pound medium shrimp, peeled and deveined

- Salt and ground black pepper, to taste

- 1/3 cup homemade chicken broth

- 2 medium zucchinis, spiralized with blade C

- ¼ cup cherry tomatoes, quartered

Direction:

1. Heat the oil in a large wok over medium heat and sauté garlic and red pepper flakes for about 1 minute.

2. Add shrimp and black pepper and cook for about 1 minute per side.

3. Add broth and zucchini noodles and cook for about 2–3 minutes.

4. Stir in tomatoes and cook for about 2 minutes.

5. Serve hot.

Nutrition:

- **Calories:** 181 Cal

- **Fat:** 18 g

- **Carbs:** 7 g

- **Protein:** 8 g

- **Fiber:** 3 g

Spinach with Cottage Cheese

Preparation Time: 15 Minutes

Cooking Time: 25 Minutes

Servings: 8

Ingredients:

- 2 (10-ounce) packages frozen spinach, thawed and drained

- 1½ cups water, divided

- ¼ cup sour cream

- 16-ounce cottage cheese, cut into ½-inch cubes

- 2 tablespoons butter

- 1 tablespoon onion, minced

- 1 tablespoon garlic, minced

- 1 tablespoon fresh ginger, minced

- 2 tablespoons tomato puree

- 2 teaspoons curry powder

- 2 teaspoons garam masala powder

- 2 teaspoons ground coriander

- 2 teaspoons ground cumin

- 2 teaspoons ground turmeric

- 2 teaspoons red pepper flakes, crushed

- Salt, to taste

Direction:

1. Place spinach, ½ cup of water, and sour cream in a blender and pulse until pureed.

2. Transfer the spinach puree into a bowl and set aside.

3. In a large non-stick wok, melt butter over medium-low heat and sauté onion, garlic, ginger, tomato puree, spices, and salt for about 2–3 minutes.

4. Add the spinach puree and remaining water and stir to combine.

5. Adjust the heat to medium and cook for about 3–5 minutes.

6. Add cottage cheese cubes and stir to combine.

7. Adjust the heat to low and cook for about 10–15 minutes.

8. Serve hot.

Nutrition:

- **Calories:** 121 Cal

- **Fat:** 12 g

- **Carbs:** 9 g

- **Protein:** 4 g

- **Fiber:** 7 g

Green Chicken Curry

Preparation Time: 15 Minutes

Cooking Time: 30 Minutes

Servings: 4

Ingredients:

- 1 pound grass-fed skinless, boneless chicken breasts, cubed

- 1 tablespoon olive oil

- 2 tablespoons green curry paste

- 1 cup unsweetened coconut milk

- 1 cup homemade chicken broth

- 1 cup asparagus spears, trimmed and cut into pieces

- 1 cup green beans, neat and cut into pieces

- Salt and ground black pepper, to taste

- ¼ cup fresh basil leaves, chopped

Direction:

1. In a wok, heat the oil over medium heat and sauté the curry paste for about 1–2 minutes.

2. Add the chicken and cook for about 8–10 minutes.

3. Add coconut milk and broth and take to a boil.

4. Adjust the heat low and cook for about 8–10 minutes.

5. Add the asparagus, green beans, salt, and black pepper, and cook for about 4–5 minutes or until desired doneness.

6. Serve hot.

Nutrition:

- **Calories:** 150 Cal

- **Fat:** 13g

- **Carbs:** 17 g

- **Protein:** 9 g

- **Fiber:** 3 g

Creamy Pork Stew

Preparation Time: 15 Minutes

Cooking Time: 95 Minutes

Servings: 8

Ingredients:

- 3 tablespoons unsalted butter

- 2½ pounds boneless pork ribs, cut into ¾-inch cubes

- 1 large yellow onion, chopped

- 4 garlic cloves, crushed

- 1½ cups homemade chicken broth

- 2 (10-ounce) cans sugar-free diced tomatoes

- 2 teaspoons dried oregano

- 1 teaspoon ground cumin

- Salt, to taste

- 2 tablespoons fresh lime juice

- ½ cup sour cream

Direction:

1. In a large heavy-bottomed pan, dissolve the butter over medium-high heat and cook the pork, onions, and garlic for about 4–5 minutes or until browned.

2. Add the broth and with a wooden spoon, scrape up the browned bits.

3. Add the tomatoes, oregano, cumin, and salt, and stir to combine well

4. Adjust the temperature to medium-low and simmer, covered for about 1½ hours.

5. Stir in the sour cream and lime juice and remove from the heat.

6. Serve hot.

Nutrition:

- **Calories:** 182 Cal

- **Fat:** 18 g

- **Carbs:** 9 g

- **Protein:** 18 g

- **Fiber:** 6 g

Salmon & Shrimp Stew

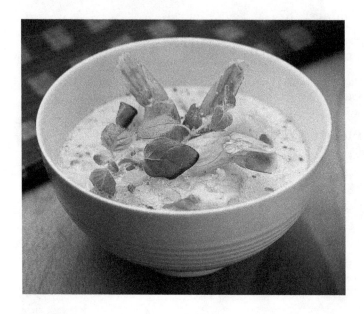

Preparation Time: 20 Minutes

Cooking Time: 25 Minutes

Servings: 6

Ingredients:

- 2 tablespoons coconut oil

- ½ cup onion, chopped finely

- 2 garlic cloves, minced

- 1 Serrano pepper, chopped

- 1 teaspoon smoked paprika

- 24 cups fresh tomatoes, chopped

- 4 cups homemade chicken broth

- 1 pound salmon fillets, cubed

- 1 pound shrimp, peeled and deveined

- 2 tablespoons fresh lime juice

- Salt and ground black pepper, to taste

- 3 tablespoons fresh parsley, chopped

Direction:

1. In a big soup pan, melt coconut oil over medium-high heat and sauté the onion for about 5–6 minutes.

2. Add the garlic, Serrano pepper, and paprika, and sauté for about 1 minute.

3. Add the tomatoes and broth and bring to a boil.

4. Adjust the heat to medium and simmer for about 5 minutes.

5. Add the salmon and simmer for about 3–4 minutes.

6. Stir in the shrimp and cook for about 4–5 minutes.

7. Stir in lemon juice, salt, and black pepper, and remove from heat.

8. Serve hot with the garnishing of parsley.

Nutrition:

- **Calories:** 168 Cal

- **Fat:** 12 g

- **Carbs:** 7.1 g

- **Protein:** 8.89 g

- **Fiber:** 3.2 g

Creamy Chicken Bake

Preparation Time: 15 Minutes

Cooking Time: 70 Minutes

Servings: 6

Ingredients:

- 5 tablespoons unsalted butter, divided

- 2 small onions, sliced thinly

- 3 garlic cloves, minced

- 1 teaspoon dried tarragon, crushed

- 8 ounces' cream cheese, softened

- 1 cup homemade chicken broth, divided

- 2 tablespoons fresh lemon juice

- ½ cup heavy cream

- 1½ teaspoons Herbs de Provence

- Salt and ground black pepper, to taste

- 4 (6-ounce) grass-fed chicken breasts

Direction:

1. Preheat the oven to 3500F.

2. Grease a 13x9-inch baking plate with 1 tablespoon of butter.

3. In a wok, melt 2 tablespoons of butter over medium heat and sauté the onion, garlic, and tarragon for about 4–5 minutes.

4. Transfer the onion mixture onto a plate.

5. In the same wok, melt remaining 2 tablespoons of butter over low heat and cook the cream cheese, ½ cup of broth, and lemon juice for about 3–4 minutes, stirring continuously.

6. 6 Stir in the cream, herbs de Provence, salt, and black pepper, and remove from heat.

7. Pour remaining broth in prepared baking dish.

8. Arrange chicken breasts in the baking dish in a single layer and top with the cream mixture evenly.

9. Bake for approximately 45–60 minutes.

10. Serve hot.

Nutrition:

- **Calories:** 129 Cal

- **Fat:** 12 g

- **Carbs:** 9 g

- **Protein:** 7 g

- **Fiber:** 5 g

Beef & Veggie Casserole

Preparation Time: 20 Minutes

Cooking Time: 55 Minutes

Servings: 6

Ingredients:

- 3 tablespoons butter

- 1 pound grass-fed ground beef

- 1 medium yellow onion, chopped

- 2 garlic cloves, chopped

- 1 cup pumpkin, peeled and chopped

- 1 cup broccoli, chopped

- 2 cups cheddar cheese, shredded

- 1 tablespoon Dijon mustard

- 6 large organic eggs

- ½ cup heavy whipping cream

- Salt and ground black pepper, to taste

Direction:

1. In a non-stick wok, melt 1 tablespoon of butter over medium heat and cook the beef for about 8–10 minutes or until no longer pink, breaking up the lumps.

2. With a positioned spoon, transfer the beef into a large bowl.

3. In the same wok, melt the remaining butter over medium heat and cook the onion and garlic for about 10 minutes, stirring frequently.

4. Add the pumpkin and cook for about 5–6 minutes.

5. Add the broccoli and cook for about 3–4 minutes.

6. Transfer the pumpkin mixture into the bowl with cooked beef and stir to combine.

7. Set aside to cool slightly.

8. Meanwhile, preheat the oven to 350°F.

9. In the bowl of beef mixture, add 2/3 of cheese and mustard and stir to combine.

10. In another mixing bowl, add cream, eggs, salt, and black pepper, and beat until well combined.

11. In a baking dish, place the beef mixture and top with egg mixture, followed by the remaining cheese.

12. Bake for approximately 25 minutes or until the top becomes golden brown.

13. Remove the baking dish from oven and set aside for about 5 minutes before serving.

14. Cut into desired-sized wedges and serve.

Nutrition:

- **Calories:** 210 Cal

- **Fat:** 18 g

- **Carbs:** 7 g

- **Protein:** 8 g

- **Fiber:** 3 g

Beef with Bell Peppers

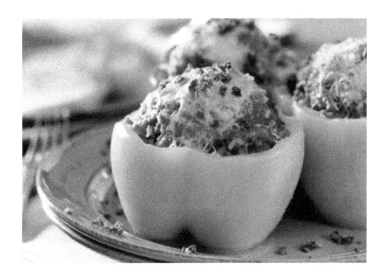

Preparation Time: 15 Minutes

Cooking Time: 10 Minutes

Servings: 4

Ingredients:

- 1 tablespoon olive oil

- 1 pound grass-fed flank steak, cut into thin slices across the grain diagonally

- 1 red bell pepper, seeded and cut into thin strips

- 1 green bell pepper, seeded and cut into thin strips

- 1 tablespoon fresh ginger, minced

- 3 tablespoons low-sodium soy sauce

- 1½ tablespoons balsamic vinegar

- 2 teaspoons Sriracha

Direction:

1. In a big non-stick wok, heat the oil over medium-high heat and sear the steak slices for about 2 minutes.

2. Add bell peppers and cook for about 2–3 minutes, stirring continuously.

3. With a slotted spoon, transfer the beef mixture into a bowl.

4. the wok, add the remaining ingredients over medium heat, and bring to a boil.

5. Cook for about 1 minute, stirring frequently.

6. Add the beef mixture and cook for about 1–2 minutes.

7. Serve hot.

Nutrition:

- **Calories:** 271 Cal
- **Fat:** 10 g
- **Carbs:** 8 g
- **Protein:** 19 g
- **Fiber:** 3 g

Coconut Keto Porridge

Preparation Time: 5 Minutes

Cooking Time: 10 Minutes

Servings: 2

Ingredients:

- 4 tbsp. of coconut cream

- 1 pinch of ground psyllium husk powder

- 1 tbsp. of coconut flour

- 1 flaxseed egg

- 1 oz. of coconut butter

Direction:

1. Toss all of the fixings together in a small pan before placing the pan on the stovetop burner set to low heat.

2. Stir the mixture as it cooks to encourage the porridge to thicken. Continue stirring until your preferred thickness is reached.

3. A small amount of coconut milk or a few berries (fresh or frozen) can also be added to taste if desired.

Nutrition:

- **Calories:** 408 Cal
- **Fat:** 20 g
- **Carbs:** 4 g
- **Protein:** 8 g
- **Fiber:** 3 g

Cream Cheese Eggs

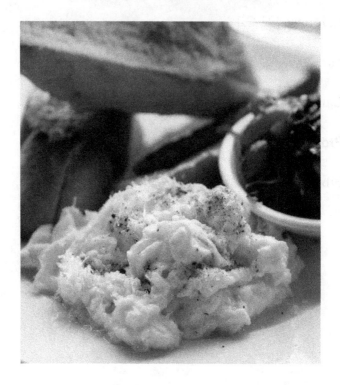

Preparation Time: 5 Minutes

Cooking Time: 5 Minutes

Servings: 2

Ingredients:

- 1 tbsp. of butter

- 2 eggs

- 2 tbsp. of soft cream cheese with chives

Direction:

1. Preheat a skillet and melt the butter.

2. Whisk the eggs with the cream cheese.

3. Add to the pan and stir until done.

Nutrition:

- **Calories:** 308 Cal

- **Fat:** 12 g

- **Carbs:** 4 g

- **Protein:** 9 g

- **Fiber:** 5 g

Creamy Basil Baked Sausage

Preparation Time: 5 Minutes

Cooking Time: 30 Minutes

Servings: 2

Ingredients:

1. 3 lb. of Italian sausage - pork/turkey or chicken

2. 8 ozs. of cream cheese

3. .25 cup of heavy cream

4. .25 cup of basil pesto

5. 8 g of mozzarella

Direction:

1. Set the oven at 400° Fahrenheit.

2. Lightly spritz a casserole dish with cooking oil spray. Add the sausage to the dish and bake for 30 minutes.

3. Combine the heavy cream, pesto, and cream cheese.

4. Pour the sauce over the casserole and top it off with the cheese.

5. Bake for another 10 minutes. The sausage should reach 160° Fahrenheit in the center when checked with a meat thermometer.

6. You can also broil for 3 minutes to brown the cheesy layer.

Nutrition:

- **Calories:** 298 Cal

- **Fat:** 17 g

- **Carbs:** 4 g

- **Protein:** 9 g

- **Fiber:** 3 g

Keto Brunch Spread

Preparation Time: 5 Minutes

Cooking Time: 20 Minutes

Servings: 4

Ingredients:

- 4 large eggs

- 24 asparagus spears

- 12 slices of sugar-free bacon

Direction:

1. Set the oven at 400° Fahrenheit.

2. Slender the asparagus about one inch from the bottoms.

3. In pairs, wrap them with one slice of bacon.

4. Firmly hold the spears in one hand as you wind the bacon slices from the bottom to the top. Pull the bacon tightly and arrange on a baking tin.

5. Repeat until you have 12 pairs.

6. Set the oven timer for 20 minutes.

7. Now, start a pot of water to a rapid boil. Place the eggs gently in the boiling water. Boil for six minutes.

8. Fill a bowl with ice water and add the eggs for another two minutes before removing the peeling from the tops/tips.

9. When the asparagus is ready, serve on a cutting board/tray. You can use an espresso cup if you don't have an egg holder to keep the eggs sitting upright.

10. Use a small spoon to scoop out the tops of the soft-boiled eggs to reveal the runny yolk.

11. Dip the asparagus into the yolks. Enjoy the egg white with some keto-friendly toast.

Nutrition:

- **Calories:** 309 Cal

- **Fat:** 10 g

- **Carbs:** 4 g

- **Protein:** 8 g

- **Fiber:** 3 g

Mushroom Omelet

Preparation Time: 5 Minutes

Cooking Time: 10 Minutes

Servings: 3

Ingredients:

- 1 oz. of butter

- 3 eggs

- 1 oz. of shredded cheese

- 3 tbsp. of yellow onion

- 3 mushrooms

Direction:

1. Whisk the eggs, salt, and pepper until frothy. Sprinkle in the spices.

2. Add the butter to a skillet. When melted, add the eggs.

3. Prepare the omelet. Once the bottom is firm, sprinkle with onions, mushrooms, and cheese.

4. Carefully remove the edges and fold the omelet in half.

5. Slide onto the plate when done to serve.

Nutrition:

- **Calories:** 309 Cal

- **Fat:** 10 g

- **Carbs:** 2 g

- **Protein:** 9 g

- **Fiber:** 4 g

1-Minute Keto Muffins

Preparation Time: 5 Minutes

Cooking Time: 35 Minutes

Servings: 3

Ingredients:

- 1 egg

- A pinch of salt

- 2 tbsp. of coconut flour

- 1 pinch of baking soda

- Butter/coconut oil (as needed)

Direction:

1. Lightly grease a large coffee mug/ramekin dish using butter or coconut

2. oil/butter.

3. Whisk all of the fixings together and cook for one minute using high for 45 seconds to one minute in the microwave. You can also bake for 12 minutes at 400° Fahrenheit in the oven.

4. Slice in half or toast and serve.

Nutrition:

- **Calories:** 172 Cal

- **Fat:** 4 g

- **Carbs:** 2 g

- **Protein:** 5 g

- **Fiber:** 2 g

Peanut Butter Protein Bars

Preparation Time: 5 Minutes

Cooking Time: 15 Minutes

Servings: 12

Ingredients:

- 1.5 cups of almond meal

- 1 cup of Keto-friendly chunky peanut butter

- 2 egg whites

- .5 cup of almonds

- .5 cup of cashews

- Also needed: baking pan

Direction:

1. Heat the oven ahead of time to reach 350° Fahrenheit.

2. Spritz a baking dish lightly with coconut or olive oil.

3. Combine all of the fixings and add them to the prepared dish.

4. Bake for 15 minutes and then cut into 12 pieces once they're cool.

5. Store in the refrigerator to keep them fresh.

Nutrition:

- **Calories:** 506 Cal

- **Fat:** 18g

- **Carbs:** 5 g

- **Protein:** 19 g

- **Fiber:** 2 g

Tuna Stuffed Avocado

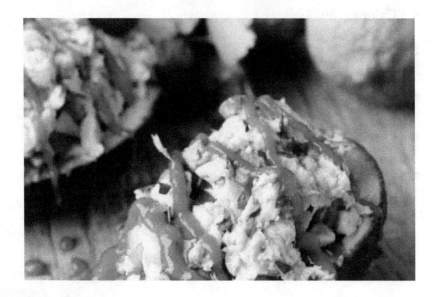

Preparation Time: 10 Minutes

Cooking Time: 0 Minutes

Servings: 4

Ingredients:

- 2 tbsp. of Greek yogurt/mayonnaise

- 5 ozs. can drained tuna

- Medium avocado

- 1 pinch of dried dill

Direction:

1. Combine the fixings (mayo, tuna, and dill).

2. Cut the avocado in half and eliminate the pit. Fill it with the salad and serve.

Nutrition:

- **Calories:** 401 Cal

- **Fat:** 20 g

- **Carbs:** 4 g

- **Protein:** 8 g

- **Fiber:** 3 g

Bacon Burger Cabbage Stir Fry

Preparation Time: 5 Minutes

Cooking Time: 20 Minutes

Servings: 10

Ingredients:

- 1 lb. of ground beef

- 1 lb. of bacon

- 1 small onion

- 3 minced cloves of garlic

- 1 lb./1 small head of cabbage

Direction:

1. Dice the bacon and onion.

2. Combine the beef and bacon in a wok or large skillet. Prepare it until done and store it in a bowl to keep warm.

3. Mince the onion and garlic. Toss both into the hot grease.

4. Slice and toss in the cabbage and stir-fry until wilted.

5. Blend in the meat and combine. Sprinkle with pepper and salt as desired.

Nutrition:

- **Calories:** 357 Cal

- **Fat:** 22 g

- **Carbs:** 6 g

- **Protein:** 20 g

- **Fiber:** 4 g

Bacon Cheeseburger

Preparation Time: 5 Minutes

Cooking Time: 0 Minutes

Servings: 12

Ingredients:

- 16 ozs. pkg. of low-sodium bacon

- 3 lbs. of ground beef

- 2 eggs

- Half of 1 medium chopped onion

- 8 ozs. of shredded cheddar cheese

Direction:

1. Fry the bacon and chop it to bits. Shred the cheese and dice the onion:-

2. Combine the mixture with the beef and blend in the whisked eggs.

3. Prepare 24 burgers and grill them the way you like them.

4. You can make a double-decker since they are small. If you like a bigger burger, you can make 12 burgers as a single-decker.

Nutrition:

- **Calories:** 489 Cal
- **Fat:** 21 g
- **Carbs:** 4 g
- **Protein:** 26 g
- **Fiber:** 3 g

Cauliflower Mac & Cheese

Preparation Time: 10 Minutes

Cooking Time: 15 Minutes

Servings: 4

Ingredients:

- 1 head of cauliflower

- 3 tbsp. of butter

- .25 cup of unsweetened almond milk

- .25 cup of heavy cream

- 1 cup of cheddar cheese

Direction:

1. Use a sharp knife to slice the cauliflower into small florets. Shred the cheese.

2. Prepare the oven to reach 450° Fahrenheit.

3. Cover a baking pan with a layer of parchment baking paper or foil.

4. Add two tablespoons of the butter to a pan and melt. Add the florets, butter, salt, and pepper together. Place the cauliflower on the baking pan and roast 10 to 15 minutes.

5. Warm up the rest of the butter, milk, heavy cream, and cheese in the microwave or double boiler. Pour the cheese over the cauliflower and serve.

Nutrition:

- **Calories:** 298 Cal

- **Fat:** 20 g

- **Carbs:** 4 g

- **Protein:** 8 g

- **Fiber:** 3 g

Mushroom & Cauliflower Risotto

Preparation Time: 15 Minutes

Cooking Time: 10 Minutes

Servings:

Ingredients:

- 1 grated head of cauliflower

- 1 cup of vegetable stock

- 9 ozs. of chopped mushrooms

- 2 tbsp. of butter

- 1 cup of coconut cream

Direction:

1. Pour the stock in a saucepan. Boil and set aside.

2. Prepare a skillet with butter and saute the mushrooms until golden.

3. Grate and stir in the cauliflower and stock.

4. Simmer and add the cream, cooking until the cauliflower is al dente. Serve.

Nutrition:

- **Calories:** 186 Cal
- **Fat:** 12 g
- **Carbs:** 4 g
- **Protein:** 9 g
- **Fiber:** 3 g

Skillet Cabbage Tacos

Preparation Time: 5 Minutes

Cooking Time: 12 Minutes

Servings: 4

Ingredients:

- 1 lb. of ground beef

- .5 cup of salsa - ex. Pace Organic

- 2 cups of shredded cabbage

- 2 tbsp. of chili powder

- .75 cup of shredded cheese

Direction:

1. Brown the beef and drain the fat. Pour in the salsa, cabbage, and seasoning.

2. Cover and lower the heat. Simmer for 10 to 12 minutes using the medium heat temperature setting.

3. When the cabbage has softened, remove it from the heat and mix in the cheese.

4. Top it off using your favorite toppings, such as green onions or sour cream, and serve.

Nutrition:

- **Calories:** 328 Cal

- **Fat:** 21 g

- **Carbs:** 4 g

- **Protein:** 18 g

- **Fiber:** 3 g

Chicken-Pecan Salad & Cucumber Bites

Preparation Time: 5 Minutes

Cooking Time: 0 Minutes

Servings: 4

Ingredients:

- 1 cucumber

- 1 cup of precooked chicken breast

- .25 cup of celery

- 2 tbsp. of mayonnaise

- .25 cup of pecans

Direction:

1. Peel and slice the cucumber into .25-inch slices. Dice the chicken and celery. Chop the pecans. Combine the pecans, chicken, mayonnaise, and celery in a salad bowl. Sprinkle with pepper and salt if desired.

2. Prepare the cucumber slices. Layer each one with a spoonful of the chicken salad. Serve.

Nutrition:

- **Calories:** 323 Cal

- **Fat:** 24 g

- **Carbs:** 5 g

- **Protein:** 4 g

- **Fiber:** 6 g

Curry Egg Salad

Preparation Time: 5 Minutes

Cooking Time: 0 Minutes

Servings: 6

Ingredients:

- 6 hard-boiled eggs

- 1 tbsp. or to taste of curry powder

- .5 cup of full-fat mayonnaise

Direction:

1. Prepare the boiled eggs by adding them into a saucepan. Pour in cold water. Turn the burner on.

2. Wait for the water to boil and set a timer for seven minutes.

3. Empty the hot water and place the eggs in a dish of cold water/ice to hinder the cooking process.

4. Once they're cool, peel and chop the eggs into small bits.

5. Combine the mayo, eggs, and curry powder.

6. Serve with a portion of chopped fresh parsley.

Nutrition:

- **Calories:** 80 Cal

- **Fat:** 5 g

- **Carbs:** 4 g

- **Protein:** 8 g

- **Fiber:** 3 g

CONCLUSION

Thank you for reading all this book!

When you are on a keto diet, your body is reducing the amount of water that you store. It can be flushing out the electrolytes that your body needs as well, and this can make you sick. Some of the ways that you can battle this is by either salting your food or drinking bone broth. You can also eat pickled vegetables.

Eat when you're hungry instead of snacking or eating constantly. This is also going to help, and when you focus on natural foods and health foods, this will help you even more. Eating foods that are processed is the worst thing you can do for fighting cravings, so you should really get into the routine of trying to eat whole foods instead.

Another routine that you can get into is setting a note somewhere that you can see it that will remind you of why you're doing this in the first place and why it's important to you. Dieting is hard, and you will have moments of weakness where you're wondering why you are doing this. Having a reminder will help you feel better, and it can really help with your perspective.

You have already taken a step towards your improvement.

Best wishes!

CPSIA information can be obtained
at www.ICGtesting.com
Printed in the USA
BVHW061544230321
603254BV00002B/43